Philosophy of Dreams

Sri Swami Sivananda

CONTENTS

Though Sri Swami Sivanandaji Maharaj is an Advaita Vedantin of Sri Sankara's School, he is unique in that in his life and teachings he synthesises the highest idealism and dynamic practical life. His "Divine Life" is ideal life, ideal and divine only because it is possible to live it here and now.

The sage, therefore, has directed the beam of his divine light on all problems that face man. Not confining himself to the exposition of philosophy and Yoga, he has enriched our literature in other fields, too, e.g., medicine, health and hygiene and even "How to Become Rich."

And now we have from his divine pen his inspiring and enlightened thoughts on one of the most interesting phenomena viz., dreams. He has viewed dreams from several angles and thrown such a flood of light on it as to expose not only its unreality, but also the unreality of the waking state. Thus the sage leads us to the Supreme Reality that alone exists.

Maha Sivaratri Day
THE DIVINE LIFE SOCIETY

Introduction

The analysis of dreams and their cause by psychoanalysts are defective. They maintain that the cause of dream creation lies in the suppressed desires of the dreamer. Can they create dreams as they like by suppressing desires? No, they cannot do that. They say that desires stimulate or help the dream creation. But they do not know what supplies the material out of which they are made and what turns the desires into actual expression, enabling the dreamer see his own suppressed desires materialised and appearing to him as real.

The desires only supply the impulse. The mind creates the dream out of the materials supplied by the experiences of the waking state. The dream creatures spring up from the bed of Samskaras or impressions in the subconscious mind. Indigestion also causes dream. The Taijasa is the dreamer. It is the waking personality that creates the dream personality. The dream personality exists as the object of the waking personality and is real only as such.

The waking and dreaming states do not exist independently side by side as real units.

Why do we dream? Various answers have been given to this question. Dreams are nothing but a reflection of our waking experience in a new form. The medical view is that dreams are due to some organic disturbances somewhere in the body, but more particularly in the stomach. Sometimes coming diseases appear in dreams.

According to Sigmund Freud all dreams without any exception are wish-fulfilment. The physical stimulus alone is not responsible for the production of dreams. The dream mechanism is very intricate. The wishes are of an immoral nature. They are revolting to the moral self, which exercises a control on their appearance. Therefore, the wishes appear in disguised forms to evade the moral censor. Very few dreams present the wishes as they really are. Dreams are partial gratification of the wishes. They relieve the mental tension and thus enable us to enjoy repose. They are safety valves to strong impulsions. You will know your animal-self in dream.

The objects which manifest during the dreaming state are often not different in many respects from those which one perceives during his waking state. During the dreaming state he talks with the members of his family and friends, eats the same food, behold rivers, mountains, motor cars, gardens, streets, ocean, temples, works in the office, answers question papers in the examination hall, and fights and quarrels with some people. This shows that man does not abandon the results of his past relation with objects when he falls asleep.

The person who experiences the three states, viz., Jagrat or waking-state, Svapna or the dreaming state, and Sushupti or deep-sleep state is called Visva in the waking state, Taijasa in the dreaming state and Prajna in the deep sleep state. When one gets up from sleep, it is Visva who remembers the experience of Prajna in deep sleep and says, "I slept soundly. I do not know anything." Otherwise remembrance of the enjoyment in deep sleep is not possible.

The reactions to dreams differ according to mental disposition, temperament and diet of the person.

All dreams are affairs of mere seconds. Within ten seconds you will experience dreams wherein the events of several years happen.

Some get dreams occasionally, while some others experience dreams daily. They can never have sleep without dreams.

The sun is the source and the temporary resting place of its rays. The rays emanate from the sun and spread in all directions at the time of sunrise. They enter into the sun at sunset, lose themselves there and come out again at the next sunrise. Even so the state of wakefulness and dream come out from the state of deep sleep and re-enter it and lose themselves there to follow the same course again.

Whatever appears in the dream world is the reproduction of the waking world. It is not only the reproduction of the objects seen, experienced or dealt with in the present life, but it may be the reproduction of objects seen, experienced or dealt with in any former life in the present world. Therefore the dream world cannot be said to be independent of the waking world.

The objects that are seen in the state of wakefulness are always seen outside the body. It is, therefore, external to the dreamer, while the dream world is always internal to the dreamer. That is the only difference between them.

During the dream state the whole wakeful world loses itself in the dream state. Therefore, it is not possible to find the distinctive features that would help the dreamer to distinguish the waking world from the dream world.

Scientists and Western philosophers draw their conclusions from the observations of their waking experience. Whereas the Vedantins utilise the experiences of the three states viz., waking, dream and deep sleep and then draw their conclusions. Hence the latter's conclusions are true, correct, perfect, full and integral, while those of the former are partial and one sided.

Certain kinds of external sounds such as the ringing of a bell, the noise of alarm-clock, knocks on the door or the wall, the blowing of wind, the drizzling of rain, the rustling of leaves, the blowing of the horn of a motor car, the cracking of the window etc., may produce in the mind of the dreamer variety of imaginations. They generate certain sensations, which increase according to the power of imagination of the sleeper and the sensitiveness of his mind. These sounds cause very elaborate dreams.

If you touch the dreamers' chest with the point of a pin, he may dream that some one has given him a severe blow on his body or stabbed him with a dagger.

The individual soul does not know that he is dreaming during his dream state and is not conscious of himself as he is bound by the Gunas of Prakriti. He passively beholds the creations of his dream mind passing before him as an effect of the workings of the impressions (Samskaras) of his waking state.

It is possible for a dreamer to remain cognisant during his dream state of the fact that he is dreaming. Learn to be the witness of your thoughts in the waking state. You can be conscious in the dream state that you are dreaming. You can alter, stop or create your own thoughts in the dream state independently. You will be able to keep awake in the dream state. If the thoughts of the waking state are controlled, you can also control the dream thoughts.

Sometimes the dreams are very interesting and turn out to be true. They foretell events. A man living in Haridwar dreamt on the first January 1947 that he will be in Benares on the night of the third January. It really turned out to be true. An officer dreams that he will be transferred to Allahabad. In the following morning he gets the transfer order. Another man dreams that he will meet with a motorcar accident on the coming Saturday. It also turns out to be true.

Profound wisdom comes through reflection on dreams. No one has known himself truly who has not studied his dreams. The study of dreams shows how mysterious is our soul. Dreams reveal to us that aspect of our nature, which transcends rational knowledge. Every dream presentation has a meaning. A dream is like a letter written in an unknown language.

Many riddles of life are solved through hints from dreams. Dreams indicate which way the spiritual life of a man is flowing. One may receive proper advice for self-correction through dreams. One may know how to act in a particular situation through dreams. The dreams point out a path unknown to the waking consciousness. Saints and sages appear in dreams during times of difficulty and point out the way.

The Vedantins study very deeply and carefully the states of dreams and deep sleep and logically prove that the waking state is as unreal as the dream state. They declare that the only difference between the two states is that the waking state is a long dream, Deergha Svapna.

So long as the dreamer dreams, dream-objects are real. When he wakes up the dream world becomes false. When one attains illumination or knowledge of Brahman, this wakeful world becomes as unreal as the dream world.

The real truth is that nobody sleeps, dreams or wakes up, because there is no reality in these states.

Transcend the three states and rest in the fourth state of Turiya, the eternal bliss of Brahman, Satchidananda Svaroopa.

Swami Sivananda

1. Songs Of Dream

Guru Guru Japna
  Aur Sab Svapna,
Guru Guru Japna
  Jagat Deergha Svapna.

Jagat Deergha Svapna
  The world is like a long dream.
Take shelter in Guru
  Everything is unreal. (Guru Guru)
Antarai

When you perceive the things in Dream
  You take them all to be real,
When you wake up and perceive
  They are all false and unreal. (Guru Guru)

The world of name and forms is like
  The dream you have during the night,
You take them all as real things,
  But they are only false and transient (Guru Guru)

The only one which really exists
  Is that God with Brahmic Splendour
Wake up, wake up, wake up to Light,
Wake up, wake up, from Maya's sleep,
  And see the things in their proper light. (Guru Guru)

2. Dream

Svapna is the dreaming state in which man enjoys the five objects of senses and all the senses are at rest and the mind alone works. Mind itself is the subject and the object. It creates all dream-pictures. Jiva is called Taijasa in this state. There is Antah-Prajna (internal consciousness). The scripture says, "When he falls asleep, there are no chariots in that state, no horses and roads, but he himself creates chariots, horses and roads."

The dreaming world is separate from the waking one. The man sleeping on a cot in Calcutta, quite healthy at the time of going to bed, wanders in Delhi as a sickly man in the dream world and vice versa. Deep sleep is separate from both the dreaming and the waking world. To the dreamer the dream world and the dream objects are as much real as the objects and experiences of the waking world. A dreaming man is not aware of the unreality of the dream world. He is not aware of the existence of the waking world, apart from the dream. Consciousness changes. This change in consciousness brings about either the waking or the dream experiences. The objects do not change in themselves. There is only change in the mind. The mind itself plays the role of the waking and the dream.
The dreamer feels that the dreams are real so long as they last, however incoherent they may be. He dreams sometimes that his head has been cut off and that he is flying in the air.

The dreamer believes in the reality of the dream as well as the different experiences in the dream. Only when he wakes up from the dream, he knows or realises that what he has experienced was mere dream, illusion and false. Similar is the case with the Jiva in the waking world. The ignorant Jiva imagines that the phenomenal world of sense-pleasure is real. But when he is awakened to the reality of things, when his angle of vision is changed, when the screen of Avidya is removed, he realises that this waking world also is unreal like the dream world.

In dream a poor man becomes a mighty potentate. He enjoys various sorts of pleasures. He marries a Maharani, lives in a magnificent palace and begets several children. He gives his eldest daughter in marriage to the son of a Maha-Raja. He goes to the Continent along with this wife and children. Then he returns and visits various places of pilgrimage. He dies of pneumonia at Benares. Within five minutes, he gets the above experiences. What a great marvel!

As in dream, so in the waking, the objects seen are unsubstantial, though the two conditions differ by the one being internal and subtle, and the other external, gross and long. The wise consider the wakeful as well as the dreaming condition as one, in consequence of the similarity of the objective experience in either case. As are dream and illusion a castle in the air, so say the wise, the Vedanta declares this cosmos to be.

Dreams represent the contraries. A king who has plenty of food, dreams that he is begging for his food in the streets. A chaste, pure aspirant dreams that he is suffering from venereal disease. A chivalrous soldier dreams that he is running from the battlefield for fear of enemy. A weak sickly man dreams that he is dead. He dreams also that his living father is dead and weeps in the night. He also experiences that he is attending the cremation of his father. Sometimes a man who lives in the city dreams that he is facing a tiger and a lion and shrieks loudly at night. He takes his pillow thinking it to be his trunk and proceeds to the Railway Station. After walking a short distance he takes it to be a dream and comes back to his house. Some people dream that they are sitting in the toilet and actually micturate in their beds.

As soon as you wake up, the dream becomes unreal. The waking state does not exist in the dream. Both dream and waking states are not present in deep sleep. Deep sleep is not present in dream and waking states. Therefore all the three states are unreal. They are caused by the three qualities: Sattva, Rajas and Tamas. Brahman or the Absolute is the silent witness of the three states. It transcends the three qualities also. It is pure bliss and pure consciousness. It is Existence Absolute.

3. Study of Dream-State

Once a disciple approached his Guru, prostrated at His Lotus Feet and with folded hands put the question:

Disciple: O My Revered Guru! Please tell me the way to cross this cycle of births and deaths.

Guru: My dear disciple! If you can understand who you are, then you can get over this cycle of births and deaths.

Disciple: O Guru! I am not so foolish as not to understand me. There is no man on earth who does not understand himself; but every one of them is having his rounds of birth and death.

Guru: No, No. You should understand the nature between the body and that person for whom this body is intended. Then only any one is said to have understood himself.

Disciple: Who is the person to whom this body belongs?

Guru: This Deha (body) belongs to the Dehi (Atman). Try to understand the true nature of the Atman.

Disciple: I do not see anybody besides this body.

Guru: When this body was asleep, who is the person who experienced your dreams? Again in deep sleep who is he that enjoyed it? When you wake up, who is he that is conscious of the world, your dreams and the soundness of the deep sleep?

Disciple: I am just beginning to have a little idea of the nature of Atman who is present in all the three states.

From the above conversation between the Guru and the disciple, it is clear that the dream and the deep sleep states are worthy of our study in order to understand the true nature of the Atman, as we already pretend to have some knowledge at least of our waking consciousness.

Dream is but a disturbance of the deep sleep and the study of the former, as to its origin, working, purpose and meaning will naturally lead us to the study of the deep sleep state also.

The best way to study a subject is to trace its history and development in the hands of eminent authors and to focus our critical faculty on what we have studied from their treaties and to rectify any omissions, when we shall have a complete and satisfactory survey of that subject.

The dream reveals within itself those unconscious mental mechanisms evolved during the course of development for the purpose of controlling and shaping the primitive instinctual self towards that form of behaviour demanded by the contemporary civilization. A working knowledge of the dream as a typical functioning of the psyche—that is, a knowledge of the dream mechanisms and of the theory of the unconscious symbolism—is therefore indispensable for dream interpretation. This knowledge may be gained intellectually from the books written by authorities on that subject, but emotional conviction is the result only of personal analytic experience. Dream should be considered as an individual psychical product from the storehouse of specific experience, which indeed the dreamer may in consciousness neither remember nor know that he knows.

In the analysis of a dream, one would say that the assimilation of knowledge of the unconscious mind through the ego is an essential part of the psychical process. The principle involved in valid explanation is the revelation of the unknown, implicit in the known in terms of the individual. This principle underlies all true dream interpretations.

The value of a dream therefore lies not only in discovering the latest material by means of the manifest content, but the language used in the narration of dream and in the giving of associations will itself help towards elucidation.

The subject of "dream" and its analysis will be, therefore, a most interesting one in understanding the true nature of the individual. We, therefore, quote in the following pages, relevant extracts from the lectures of Sigmund Freud, the famous authority on that subject and will evolve it further, if necessary, by the help of the knowledge we get from the Indian Sages and Seers.

4. Dream Philosophy

Certain Karmas are worked out in dreams also. A King experienced a dream in which he acts the part of a beggar and suffers the pangs of starvation. Certain evil Karmas of the King are purged out in this experience.

If a man is not able to become a king on account of evil influence of some planets, he plays the part of a king in his dream. His strong desire materialises in the dream state.

One derives more pleasure in dream than in the waking state when he experiences pleasant dreams because the mind works more freely in dream.

If you have made arrangements to go to Bombay in the morning of 30th April, you may experience a dream on the night of 29th itself that you are purchasing a ticket at the station and entering the train and some friends have come on the platform of Bombay station to receive you. The strong thoughts of the waking state find expression at once in the dreaming state.

When a strong desire is not gratified in the waking state, you obtain its gratification in dream. The mind has more freedom in the dreaming state. The mind is then like a furious elephant let loose.

5. *Philosophy of Dream*

I

One dreams many things that are never to be experienced in this life such as "He dreams he is flying in the air."

A dream is not an entirely new experience, because most often it is the memory of past experiences.

In the waking state the light of the self is mixed up with the functions of the organs, intellect, mind, external lights etc. In dreams the self becomes distinct and isolated as the organs do not act and the lights such as the sun that help them are absent.

The dreamer is not affected by whatever result of the good and evil he sees in the dream state. No one regards himself a sinner on account of the sins committed in dreams. People who have heard of them do not condemn or shun them. Hence he is not touched by them.

The dreamer only appears to be doing things in dream but actually there is no activity The Sruti says, "He sees to be enjoying himself in the company of women." (Bri. Up. IV. iii. 13.) He who described his dream experiences uses the words 'as if'; "I saw today as if a herd of elephants was running." Therefore the dreaming self has no activity in dreams.

An action is done by the contact of the body and the senses, which have form with something else that has form. We never see a formless thing being active. The Self is formless. Therefore it is not attached. As this Self is unattached, it is untouched by what it beholds in dreams. Hence we cannot ascribe activity to it, as activity proceeds from the contact of the body and the organs. There is no contact for the Self, because this infinite Self is unattached. Therefore it is immortal.

Doctors say, "Do not wake him up suddenly or violently", because they see that in dreams the self goes out of the body of the waking state through the gates of the organs and remains isolated outside. If the self is violently aroused it may not find those gates of the organs. If he does not find the right organ the body becomes difficult to doctor. The self may not get back to those gates of the organs, things which it sent out taking the shining functions of the latter, or it may misplace those functions. In that case defects such as blindness and deafness may result. The doctor may find it difficult to treat them.

II

Dreams are due to mental impressions (Vasanas) received in the waking state. The consciousness in a dream depends on the previous knowledge acquired in the wakeful state.

The dreams have the purpose of either cheering or saddening and frightening the sleeper, so as to requite him for his good and evil deeds. His Adrishta thus furnishes the efficient cause of the dreams.

Even in the state of dream the instruments of the self are not altogether at rest, because scripture states that even then it is connected with Buddhi (intellect). "Having become a dream, together with Buddhi it passes beyond this world."

Smriti also says, "When the senses being at rest, the mind not being at rest, is occupied with the objects, know that state to be a dream."

Scripture says that desires etc. are modifications of the mind (Bri, Up. I-v-3). Desires are observed in dreams. Therefore, the self wanders about in dreams together with the mind only.

The scripture in describing our doings in dreams qualifies them by an 'as it were'. "As it were rejoicing together with women, or laughing as it were, or seeing terrible sights" (Bri. Up. IV-iii-13). Ordinary people also describe the dreams in the same manner. "I ascended as it were the summit of a mountain, I saw a tree, as it were".

Dream creation is unreal. Reality implies the factors of time, space and causation. Further, reality cannot be sublated or stultified. Dream creation has not got these traits.

Dream is called 'Sandhya' or the intermediate state because it is midway between waking and the deep sleep state, between the Jagrat and the Sushupti.

III

Dreams, though of a strange and illusory nature, are a good index of the high or low spiritual and moral condition of the dreamer. He, who has a pure heart and untainted character, will never get impure dreams. An aspirant who is ever meditating will dream of his Sadhana and his object of meditation. He will do worship of the Lord and recite His name and Mantra even in dream through the force of Samskara.

6. Who is it That Dreams?

If you ask any man in this world, "Who is it that wakes up? Who is it that dreams? And who is it that sleeps?" He will answer, "It is I that wake up; it is I that dream; it is I that sleep." If you ask him "What is this I?" he will say, "this body is the 'I'." He will tell you that it is the body that sleeps. When the brain is tired or exhausted, it is the body that sleeps; when the brain is disturbed, it is the body that dreams; and when the brain is refreshed, it is the body that wakes up after sound sleep.

A psychologist who has made a special study of the mind will say that the mind, which has its seat in the brain, is the 'I'. He says that the mind is inseparable from the brain and it perishes along with the physical body.

The metaphysicians and the spiritualists hold that the mind continues to exist somewhere after the death of the body. According to psychologists, metaphysicians and spiritualists it is the mind that wakes up, dreams and sleeps and this mind is the 'I'.

A Theologist says that there is a soul which is quite independent of the body and the mind and it is this soul that wakes up, dreams and sleeps and the soul is the 'I'. This soul enters another body in accordance with the law of Karma.

A Vedantin says that neither this body nor the mind nor the soul is the 'I'. There is one pure consciousness or Atman in all beings which is Infinite, Eternal, all-pervading, self-existent, self-luminous and self-contained which is partless, timeless, spaceless, birthless, and deathless. This is the real 'I'. This 'I' never wakes, dreams or sleeps. It is always the seer or the silent witness (Sakshi) of the three states of waking, dreaming and sleeping. It is the Turiya or the fourth state. It is the state that transcends the three states.

It is the false or relative 'I' called Ahamkara or ego or that Jiva that wakes up, dreams and sleeps. The waker, the dreamer and the sleeper are all changing personalities and unreal.

The real self, the real 'I' never wakes up, dreams and sleeps. From the point of the Absolute Truth or Paramartha Satta no one wakes up, dreams and sleeps.

7. Lord Creates Dream Objects

(Another view)

Some Indian philosophers hold that the creation of chariots etc. in the dream is verily by the Lord and not by the human self. The dream objects are created by the Lord as fruition of the minor works of the Jiva. In order to reward the soul for very minor Karmas, the Lord creates the dreams.

The followers of one Sakha, namely the Kathakas, state in their text that the Supreme Lord is alone the Creator of all Karmas in the dream state for the dreamers (Katha Up. V-8).

"He, the Highest Person, who is awake in us when we are asleep, shaping one lovely sight after another, that indeed is the Bright, that is Brahman, that alone is called the Immortal. All worlds are contained in Him, and no one goes beyond Him. This is that."

Maya or the will of the Lord is the only means through which He creates dream objects. They are not made of objective matter (gross elements) because they are not perceptible to all persons, but are seen only by the dreamer.

He who can cause the bondage and release of the soul can easily bring about the dream and its withdrawal for the soul. There is nothing wonderful in it. Kurma Purana says: "It is He (the Lord) who makes the soul perceive the dream creation etc. and it is He who hides them from his view; for on His will the bondage and release of the soul depend."

8. Prophetic Dreams

Sometimes dreams are prophetic of future good and bad fortune. The scripture teaches, "When a man engaged in some work undertakes for a special wish, sees in his dreams a woman, he may infer success from that dream vision". "Then having washed the Mantha vessel which should be either of bell-metal or of wood, let him lie down behind the fire on a skin or on a bare ground silently and singly. If in his dreams he sees a woman, let him know this is an omen that his sacrifice has been successful". (Chh. Up. V-2-8-9).

Other scriptural passages declare that certain dreams indicate speedy death e.g. "If he sees a black man with black teeth, that man will kill him" (Kaushitaki Brahmana.)

Those who also understand the science of dreams hold the opinion that the dream of riding on an elephant and the like is lucky; while it is unlucky to dream of riding on a donkey.

Lord Siva taught Visvamitra in dream the Mantra called "Ramaraksha". He exactly wrote it out in the morning when he awoke from sleep.

Works of genius like poems etc. are found in dreams. Remedies for diseases are prescribed in the dream. Sometimes the exact object seen in dreams is seen afterwards in waking state.

Vyasa and other sages who know the science of dreams say, "Whatever a Brahmin or a God, a bull or a king may tell a person in dreams will doubtless prove true".

Ramanuja holds, "Because the images of a dream are produced by the Highest Lord Himself, therefore, they have prophetic significance."

9. Spiritual Enlightenment Through Dreams

"He who is happy within, who rejoices within, and who is illumined within, that Yogi attains absolute freedom or Moksha, himself becoming Brahman." (Gita: V-24.) The highest spiritual knowledge is Knowledge of the Self. He who has known himself, rather his self, for him nothing remains to be known. The wisest of the Western philosophers Socrates, gave the highest and the best of his teachings to his disciples in the injunction "Know Thyself". The Indian saints likewise gave their highest teaching in the form known as Adhyatma-Vidya or Self-Knowledge.

Knowledge of the Self, which has been called the supreme knowledge by the wise men of all ages, has seldom been recognised as a mystery by the ordinary man. He seems to know himself so well that he does not think it even necessary to reflect upon himself. Not only does the uneducated illiterate person think it useless to reflect upon himself, but the highly cultured modern man also thinks in the same way. The greater the advancement of science and learning, the less we find in the modern man a desire to know himself.

There are two opposite reasons that lead a man not to reflect upon himself: first, he thinks that he knows the self too well, secondly he thinks it useless to think about himself, because the true nature of the self can never be known. Some think that thinking about oneself is a morbid mentality. This is a form of introversion from which one has to free oneself as soon as possible. The study of dreams is corrective to such an erroneous view.

There was a time when psychologists thought, the less we thought about our dreams, the better. The psychologists who take consciousness to be an epi-phenomenon still hold the same view. Seashore, for instance, thinks that it is only abnormal people who think too much of their dreams, and that thinking too much about dreams leads to abnormalities. There is much in the waking life to be attended to and he who spends his time in thinking about his dreams is missing so much of his waking life and this contributes to his own failure in life.

Now Psychology, however, has changed this point of view. It shows that deepest wisdom comes through reflection on dreams. No one has known himself truly, who has not studied his dreams. The study of dreams at once shows what a great mystery our soul is, and that this mystery is not altogether insoluble, as some metaphysicians supposed. Dreams reveal to us that aspect of our nature which transcends rational knowledge. That in the most rational and moral man there is an aspect of his being which is absurd and immoral, one knows only through the study of one's dreams. All our pride of nationality and morality melts into nothingness as soon as we reflect upon our dreams.

There is logic in our dreams or rather the logic of our waking consciousness is just like the dream logic. The great philosopher Hegel constructed his logic without taking into account what the dream logic has to reveal. Now logic, which at the same time claims to be a system of Metaphysics, cannot be complete without taking into account the absurd constructions of dream experience. Logic is only a tool of intellect, which enables it to deal with the waking experience alone. This fact is revealed to us through the study of our dreams. The real must transcend all logical categories; or the categories by which it can be comprehended have to be such as will not only suffice to catch the waking experience but the dream experience too. This simply means that it should be broad enough to comprehend both the conscious and the unconscious life of a man. To conceive of such a category cannot be the work of waking consciousness. Such a category must necessarily transcend both the waking and the dream consciousness. Thus we are lead to the necessity of intuition or a logical thought to comprehend Reality, when we begin reflecting upon our dreams.

The modern study of dreams shows that they are not meaningless presentations. Every dream presentation has a meaning. A dream is like a letter written in an unknown language. To a man who does not know the Chinese, a letter written in that language is a meaningless scroll. But to one who knows that language it is full of most valuable information. It may be the letter calls for immediate action; or it may contain words of consultation to one suffering from dejection. It may be a letter of threat or it may speak of love. These meanings are there only to one who would care to attend to the letter and would try to decipher it. But alas! How few of us try to understand these messages from the deep unseen ocean of our own Consciousness!

Why do we dream? Various answers have been given to this question. According to the most popular scientific view, dreams are nothing but a repetition of our waking experiences in a new form. A more thoughtful view regards them as productions of an organic disturbance somewhere in the body, but more particularly in the stomach. To this view medical men stick more tenaciously than any other people. Sometimes coming diseases appear in dreams. During an illness dreams are generally more horrible than they are in the healthy condition of the body. These are all scientific theories of dreams. We have here out of account the unscientific theories, e.g. that dreams are premonitions or that gods or demons or spirits produce dreams, or that the soul goes out to a sojourn in dreams etc.

The scientific theories have been very thoroughly exposed by Dr. Sigmund Freud in his Interpretation of Dreams. No physical stimulus, whether it is inside or outside the body, no experience of the waking or sleeping state can explain the presentation of the actual dream content. The same stimulus, namely the chime of an alarm timepiece produced three different kinds of dreams to Hidetrant at different times. Why should it be so if the physical stimulus alone is responsible for the production of dreams?

According to Freud all dreams, without any exception, are wish fulfilment. The wishes are actually of an immoral nature. They are revolting to the moral self, which exercises a control on their appearance. Hence to evade this moral censor the wishes appear in disguised forms. The dream mechanism is very intricate. Very few dreams present the wishes as they really are. Dreams are partial gratification of the wishes. They relieve the mental tension, and thus enable us to enjoy repose. They are safety valves to strong impulsions. Dreams do not disturb sleep but rather protect it. The irrationality and the immorality of dreams make the morality and rationality of our waking life possible.

The above statement of Freud shows that we know our animal self in dream. But he does not say anything about the spiritual life being expressed in dream. This, it seems, has been done by Jung. According to Jung, a dream is not causally determined as was supposed by Freud, but it is teleologically determined. The repressed wishes alone do not explain all our dreams. A dream presents a demand to our waking consciousness. If rightly interpreted, it shows the way to be at peace with ourselves. The dreams of the neurotics not only reveal the repressed contents but they also suggest remedies for the cure. A series of dreams sometimes occur to a patient, which reveal the way to cure.

The dream consciousness is superior to the waking consciousness in many respects. Many puzzles of life are solved through hints from dreams. All dreams, according to Adler, are anticipatory in character. They show which way the spiritual life of a man is flowing. To know the actual flow is necessary to correct possible errors. Dreams help us to discover the lifeline of the individual and help us to give him proper advice for self-correction.

Thus, through dreams one may know how one ought to act in a particular situation. The dreams point out a path unknown to the waking consciousness. Saints and sages appear in dreams at times of difficulty and show the way. The more one follows the dream intuitions, the clear they become.

10. *Waking as a Dream*

In both states—waking and dreaming—objects are "Perceived", i.e., are associated with subject-object relationship. This is the similarity between the two.

The only difference between the two states is that the objects in dream are perceived in the space within the body, whereas in the waking condition they are seen in the space outside the body. The fact of "being seen" and their consequent illusoriness are common to both states.

The illusion of both the states is established by their "being seen" as "object", other then the self, thus creating a difference in existence. Anything that is "perceived" is unreal, for perception presupposes relation and relation is non-eternal, for the relations of the waking state are contradicted by those of dream and vice versa. As duality is unreal, all objects must be unreal.

As long as the dream lasts, waking is unreal; as long as waking lasts, dream is unreal. The reality of the one is dependent on the reality of the other. But dream is proved to be unreal; hence waking also is unreal.

Dream-relations are contradicted by waking-relations. Waking relations are contradicted by Super-consciousness which is uncontradicted. Non-contradiction is the test of reality.

That which persists forever is real. That which does not and which has a beginning and an end is unreal. Dream and waking have both a beginning and an end. But it may be contented that one thing exists as the cause of the other in the beginning. But as causality itself is baseless, a thing cannot exist as the cause of another. That which has a beginning and an end is changeable and hence non-eternal and unreal, for change implies non-existence in the beginning or at an end. Hence all perceived objects are unreal.

As the objects of the waking state do not work in dream, they are unreal. As the objects of the dream do not work in the waking state, they are unreal. Hence everything is unreal. One who eats belly-full during the waking state feels hungry in the dream state and vice versa. Things are real only in their own realms and not always. That which is not always real is unreal, for reality is everlasting.

The perception of an object is unreal, because the objects are creations of the mind. An object has got a particular form, because the mind believes it to be so. In fact, the objects of both the dreaming and the waking states are unreal. An object lasts only as long as the particular mental condition cognising the object lasts. When there is a different mental condition altogether, the objects also change. Hence all objects are unreal.

Both in the dream and in the waking stale, the internal perceptions are unreal and the objects of external perception appear to be real.

If in the waking state we make a distinction of real and unreal, in dream also we do the same thing. In dream also objects of internal cognition, are unreal. Dream is as real as the waking state. But since dream is proved to be unreal, waking also must be unreal. Dream is unreal only from the standpoint of waking, and equally so is waking to the dreamer. From the standpoint of True Wisdom, waking is as unreal as dream.

11. *The Unreality of Imagination*

Through the play of the mind in dreams and deliriums nearness appears as a great distance and a great distance appears as proximity. Through the force of the mind a great cycle of time appears as a moment and a moment appears as a great cycle. The unreal world appears as real whereas it is in reality a long dream arisen in our mind. This world is nothing but a long dream. The mind sports and creates an illusion. Through the play of the mind the dream-world appears as real. The following story will illustrate this fact.

Lavana was a king of the country of Uttara Pandava. He was once seated on his throne. All his ministers and officers were present. There appeared at this time a Siddha or a magician. He bowed down to the king and said, "O Lord! Deign to behold my wonderful feats." The Siddha waved his bunch of peacock feathers. The king had the following experiences. A messenger from the king of Sindhu entered the court with a horse like that of Indra and said, "O Lord! My master has made a present of this horse to you." The Siddha requested the king to mount upon the horse and ride it at his pleasure. The king stared at the horse and entered into a state of trance for two hours. Afterwards there was relaxation of rigidity of his body. The king's body fell on the ground after some time. The courtiers lifted the body. The king gradually came to consciousness. The ministers and the courtiers said to the king: "What is the matter with your majesty?" The king said: "The Siddha waved his bunch of peacock's feathers. I saw a horse before me. I mounted on the horse and rode in a desert in the hot sun. My tongue was parched. I was quite fatigued. Then I reached a beautiful forest. While I was riding on the horse, a creeper encircled my neck and the horse ran away. I was rocking to and fro in the air during the whole of the night with the creeper encircling my neck. I was shivering with extreme cold.

"The day dawned and I saw the sun. I cut the creeper that encircled my neck. I then beheld an outcaste girl carrying some food and water in her hands. I was very hungry and asked her to give me some food. She did not give me anything. I followed her closely for a long time. She then turned to me and said: "I am a Chandala by birth. If you promise to marry me in my own place before my parents and live with me there, I will give you what I have in my hand this very moment." I agreed to marry her. She then gave me half of the food. I ate the food and drank the beverage of Jambu fruits.

"Then she took me to her father and asked his permission to marry me. He consented. Then she took me to her abode. The father of the girl killed monkeys, cows and pigs for flesh and dried them on the strings of nerves. A small shed was erected. I had then my seat on a big plantain leaf. My squint-eyed mother-in-law then looked at me with her blood-red eyeballs and said, "Is this our would-be son-in-law?"

"The marriage festivities began with great éclat. My father-in-law presented me clothes and other articles. Toddy and meat were freely distributed. The meat-eating Chandalas beat their drums. The girl was given to me in marriage. I was named as 'Pushta.' The wedding festival lasted for seven days. A daughter was first born of this union. She brought forth again a black boy in the course of three years. She again gave birth to a daughter. I became an old Chandala with a large family and lived for a long time. Children are a source of grief. Miseries of human beings which arise out of passion take the form of a child. My body became old and emaciated on account of family cares and worries. I had to undergo pain through heat and cold in the dreary forest. I was clad in old ragged clothes. I carried loads of firewood on my head. I was exposed to the chill winds. I had to live upon the roots. I thus spent sixty years of my life as if they were so many Kalpa-ages of long duration. There was severe famine. Many died of starvation. Some of my relatives left the place.

"I and my wife left the country and walked in the hot sun. I carried two children on my shoulders and third on my head. I walked a long distance and then arrived at the fringe of a forest. We all took a little rest under a big palmyra tree. My wife expired on account of long travel in the hot sun. My younger son Pracheka rose up and stood before me and said with tears gushing out of his eyes: "Papa, I am hungry. Give me immediately some meat and drink or else I will die." He repeatedly said with tears in his eyes that he was dying of hunger. I was then moved by paternal affection. I was very much afflicted at heart. I was not able to bear the distress. Then I made up my mind to put an end to my life by falling into fire. I collected some wood, heaped them together and set fire to them. I stood up to jump into the fire when I fell down from throne and woke up. I now find myself as the king Lavana once again and not as a Chandala."

This story illustrates the heterogeneous actions of the mind. The experiences of the state of trance or delirium, the experiences in the waking state and those in dream are all similar. The Samskaras are ingrained in the mind equally in all the states of consciousness. The misery of Samsara is equally felt in all the states of the mind when it is vigorously working. Whatever we see is only a manifestation of the mind. It is quite illusory. Time is but a mode of mind. Centuries are passed for but five minutes and vice versa. Within two hours, king Lavana had experienced such a diverse life of sixty years.

None can say whether his life as king was true or as Chandala. Whether this is a dream or that is a dream we cannot say. Instead of thinking that the king dreamt of a life as Chandala, we can as well consider that a real Chandala dreamt that he was king Lavana. Both are unintelligible and unreal modes of imagination. Our whole life on earth is a similar play of imagination. Our states of consciousness contradict themselves when we try to reconcile them. We cannot say whether we are dreaming or waking. To us every state of imagination seems to be real. We may be in this world building castles in the air while sleeping on the bed in some other world. Nothing can be given as a proof for the reality of the world in which we live. If all of us now experience a common world it may be due to an apparent accident in the similarity of the states of consciousness in us. And moreover there is no guarantee that all of us look at the world in the same fashion. The world changes from person to person and to the same person at different conditions of the mind. This is the state of dream and waking.

We are so much engaged with the present state of the mind and so attached to the persisting condition of imagination, that nothing but the actual present seems to be real. We forget the past and ignore the future. We think now that the dream of yesterday is a falsity. And in the state of dream we apply the same conviction to the waking state also. Are we not mere slaves of imagination? Our individual life is thus proved to be a fallacy and a vile creature of the modes of imagination, which is itself an illusion!

12. Why Jagrat is a Dream?

Jagrat Avastha is waking consciousness. You perceive, feel, think, know and you are conscious of the external sense-universe. The organs of hearing and sight are very vigilant. The organ of sight is more active than the ear. It rushes headlong over forms (Rupa), various types of beauty, through force of habit. The Abhimani (person thinking upon) of Jagrat state is termed as Visva. He identifies himself with the physical body. Visva is Vyasthi (individual) Abhimani. The Samasthi Abhimani (cosmic) is Virat. Visva is microcosm (Kshudra Brahmanda). Virat is macrocosm (Brahmanda). Vyasthi is single. Samashti is sum-total. A single matchstick is Vyasthi. A matchbox is Samasthi. A single house is Vyashti. A village is Samasthi. A single mango tree is Vyasthi. A grove of mango-trees is Samasthi. Ear and eye are the avenues of sense-knowledge in the Jagrat State.

The mind creates the dream-world out of the experience and Samskaras of the waking consciousness.

Dream is a reproduction of the experiences of the physical consciousness with some modifications. The mind weaves out the dream creatures out of the material supplied from waking consciousness. In dream the subject and object are one. The perceiver and the perceived are one in this state. The Abhimani of Svapna Avastha is Taijasa. Taijasa is a Vyasthi Abhimani. The Samasthi Abhimani is Hiranyagarbha, the first-born.

In the Jagrat state there are two kinds of knowledge, viz., Abijna or Abijna Jnana and Pratibijna or Pratibijna Jnana. Abijna is knowledge through perception. You see a tree. You know: "This is a tree". This is Abijna. Pratibijna is recognition. Here something previously observed is recognised in some other thing or place, as when, for instance, the generic character of a cow which was previously observed in the black cow again presents itself to consciousness in the grey cow or Mr. Radhakrishnan whom I first saw in Benares in 1922 again appears before me in Calcutta in 1932. There are cases of recognition where the object previously observed again presents itself to our senses. There is a Samskara in the mind of object, time and place. When I recognised Mr. Radhakrishnan in Calcutta, I omitted the previous place Benares where I saw him for the first time and the time also 1922 and I took into consideration the present place Calcutta and the present time 1932. This is knowledge through Pratibijna. In Abijna, there is no Antahkarana Samskaras. There is knowledge through mere sense-contact with the object.

When you take a retrospective view of your life in college when you are 60 years of age, it is all a dream to you. Is it not so, my friends? The future also will turn out to be so. There is only the present, which on account of the force of strong Samskaras through repetition of actions and Dhrida (strong) Vasanas appears to be real for an Aviveki (a man of non-discrimination) only. The past is a dream. The future is a dream. The solid present is also a dream. When you are alone at Allahabad for a month, you have entirely forgotten all about Chennai, your affairs, family, children etc. You have only Allahabad Samskaras. For the time being Chennai is out of your mind. There is only Allahabad in your mind. When you return again to Chennai, Allahabad affairs entirely disappear from the mind after some time. When you are in Allahabad, Chennai is a dream to you, and when you are in Chennai, Allahabad is a dream. World is a mere Samskara in the mind. For a worldly man with a gross mind full of passions this world is a solid reality.

According to Gaudapada, Dada-Guru of Sri Sankaracharya, the Jagrat Avastha is exactly a dream without any difference. Some saints say that the waking state is a long dream (Deerga Svapna). An objector says: "In Jagrat state we see the same objects in the same place as soon as we wake up (Desa Kala), whereas in dreams, we do not see again the same objects. We see different things daily. How do you account for this?"

Even in dreams sometimes we see same objects repeatedly on different occasions.

Every moment the whole world is changing. You do not see the same world every day. Young people become old. The molecules of the body are changing every second. Mind also changes every moment. Trees and all objects are continually changing. The water that you see in the Ganga at 6 a.m. is not the same when you see at 6.05 a.m. When a wick in the hurricane lamp is burning, you see the light but the wick is ever changing. There are continual changes in sun, moon, stars etc. The world is stationary for people of gross minds (Sthula Buddhi). A man of Sukshma (subtle) intellect does not see the same world every day. He witnesses changes—changes in every second and sees daily a new world. Therefore the waking consciousness also is a dream. Just as the dream becomes false as soon as you wake up, the Jagrat consciousness becomes a dream when you get Viveka and Jnana. Science tells you that the world is a mass of electrons that are in constant rotation and change.

An objector again says: "We remember the events, the persons, the places etc., in Jagrat Avastha. In dream we do not remember. How do you explain this?"

In Svapna or dream state there is Rajo Guna Pradhana. Rajo Guna predominates. In Jagrat state, Sattva Guna predominates. That is the reason why you have no remembrance in dream.

As soon as you wake up, the dreams turn out to be false. So long as you are dreaming, every thing is real to you. This world, the waking consciousness, becomes a dream when you get Jnana. Therefore Jagrat is termed as a dream. This appears to be paradoxical but it is not so. Think well.

In prophetic dreams the materials come from the Karana Sarira or seed body (causal body), the storehouse of Samskaras.

Readers are earnestly requested to go through very carefully Mandukya Upanishad with Gaudapada's Karika either in Sanskrit or English translation. The dream problem is very elaborately dealt with cogent argument.

"When I consider the matter carefully, I do not find a single characteristic by means of which I can certainly determine whether I am awake or whether I dream. The visions of

a dream and the experiences of my waking state are so much alike that I am completely puzzled and I do not really know that I am not dreaming at this moment." (Descartes: Meditations P. I.)

Pascal is right when he asserts that if the same dream comes to us every night we should be just as much occupied by it as by the things which we see every day. To quote his words, "If an artisan were certain that he would dream every night for fully 12 hours that he was a king, I believe that he would be just as happy as a king who dreams every night for 12 hours that he is an artisan".

In dream the seer and the seen are one. The mind creates the bee, flower, mountain, horses, rivers, etc., in the dream. The dream objects are not independent of the mind. They have no separate existence apart from the mind. So long as the dream lasts, the dream creatures will remain just as the milkman remains so long as the milking goes on. (The dream is quite real when the man is dreaming). Whereas in the Jagarat state the object exists independent of the mind. The objects of the waking experiences are common to us all, while those of dreams are the property of the dreamer.

Jacob puts Gaudapada's arguments in the following syllogistic form: "Things seen in the waking state are not true: this is proposition (Pratijna); because they are seen, this is reason (Hetu); just like things seen in a dream, this is the instance (Drishtanta); as things seen in the dream are not true, so the property of the being seen belongs in like manner to things seen in the waking state; this is the application of the reason (Hetupanyaya); therefore things seen in the waking state are also untrue; this is the conclusion.

Gaudapada establishes the unreal Character of the world of experience:

1. By its similarity to dream state;

2. By its presented or objective character;

3. By the unintelligibility of the relations which organise it; and

4. By its non-persistence for all time.

13. Waking Experience Has Relative Reality

I

Waking experience is like dream experience
When judged from the absolute standpoint.
But it has Vyavaharika-Satta
Or relative reality.
Dream is Pratibhasika-Satta
Or apparent reality.
Turiya or Brahman is Paramarthika-Satta
Or Absolute Reality.
Waking is reality more real than dreaming.
Turiya is more real than waking.
From the point of view of Turiya,
Both waking and dreaming are unreal.
But waking, taken by itself,
In relation to dream experience,
Has greater reality than dream.
To a certain extent,
As Turiya is to waking,
Waking is to dream.
Waking is the reality behind dream;
Turiya is the reality behind waking.
Dream is not dream to the dreamer.
Only by one who is awake
Dream is known to be a dream.
Similarly, waking appears to be real
To one who is still in the waking state.
Only to one who is in Turiya
Waking is devoid of reality.
Waking is Deergha-Svapna,
A long dream, as contrasted with
The ordinary dream which is short.

II

Waking is a part of Virat-Consciousness,
Though, in waking, due to ignorance,
The Virat is not directly realised.
Waking is the connecting link
Between Visva and Virat.
Man reflects over the world and the Reality
When he is awake
And when his consciousness is active.

In dream, the intellect and the will
Are incapacitated due to Avidya
And deliberate contemplation becomes impossible.
The Visva or the Jiva in the waking state
Is possessed of intelligence and free will.
The Taijasa or the Jiva in the dreaming state
Is destitute of such powers of free thinking.
Dream experience is the result of
Impressions of waking experience;
Whereas, waking experience is independent of
Dream experience and its effects.
There is a kind of order or system
In the waking experiences,
At least, more than in dream.
Every day the same persons and things
Become the objects of waking experience.
There is a definite remembrance of
Previous days' experiences and of
Survival and continuity of personality
In waking experience.
The consciousness of this continuity,
Regularity and unity
Is absent in dream,
Dream is not well ordered,
While waking is comparatively systematic.

III

There are degrees of reality
In the experiences of the individual.
The three main degrees are
Subjective, Objective and Absolute.
Dream experience is subjective.
Waking experience is objective.
The realisation of Atman or Brahman
Is experience of the absolute Reality.
The individual is the subjective being
In comparison with the objective world.
The subject and the object have equal reality,
Though both these are negated in the Absolute.
The objective world is the field of waking experience
And, therefore, waking is relatively real.
But, dream is less real than waking
In as much as the direct contact
With the external world of waking experience

Is absent in dream.
Though there is an external world in dream also,
Its value is less than that of the world in waking.
Though the form of the dream world agrees with
That of the waking world,
In quality the dream world
Is lower than the waking world.
Space, time, motion and objects,
With the distinction of subject and object,
Are common to both waking and dreaming.
Even the reality they present
At the time of their being experienced
Is of a similar nature.
But, the difference lies in
The degree of reality manifested by them.
The Jiva feels that it is in a higher order of truth
In waking than in dreaming.

IV

The argument that is advanced
To prove the unreality of waking
Is that waking also is merely mind's play
Even as dream is mind's imagination.
But, the objects seen in dream
Are not imaginations of the dream subject
Which itself is one of the imaginary forms
That are projected in dream,
The dream subject is not in any way
More real than the dream objects.
They both have equal reality
And are equally unreal.
The dream subject and the dream object
Are both imaginations of the mind of Visva
Which synthesises the subject and objects in dream.
In like manner, the waking individual
Is not the cause of the objects seen by it,
For both these belong to the same order of reality.
Neither of them is more real than the other.
The virtues and the defects that characterise things
Are present in all subjects and objects
That are experienced in the waking state.
The subject and the objects in waking
Are both effects of the Cosmic Mind
Which integrates all the contents of the universe.

The Cosmic Mind has greater reality
Than the individual mind.
Thus the waking state is relatively
More real than the dreaming state.

V

It cannot be said that
Taijasa is related to Hiranyagarbha
In the same way as
Visva is related to Virat.
Taijasa has a negative experience
Characterised by fickleness, absence of clearness,
Lack of will power and cloudedness of intelligence.
To express with certain reservations,
The relation of Taijasa to Hiranyagarbha
Is something like that of minus two to plus two:
Whereas, Visva is to Virat
As minus one is to plus one.
As minus one has greater positive value
Than minus two,
And the distance between minus two and plus two
Is greater than that between
Minus one and plus one,
Visva has greater relative value than Taijasa,
And is more intimately connected with Virat
Than Taijasa with Hiranyagarbha.
Taijasa and Prajna are respectively
The parts of Hiranyagarbha and Isvara
Only as limited reflections with negative values
And not positively and qualitatively.
Otherwise Isvara would have been only
A huge mass of ignorance,
As he is depicted as the collective totality
Of all Prajnas whose native experience is a state of sleep
Where ignorance covers the existing consciousness.
Prajna and Isvara are like minus three and plus three,
And their relation is quite obvious.
As when a man stands on a river bank
And looks at his own reflection below,
That which is highest appears as lowest—
The original head is farthest from the reflected head,—
That which is lowest appears as highest—
The original feet are nearest to the reflected feet,—
In the same manner, Isvara,

Who is the highest among the manifestations of reality
And is omniscient and omnipotent
Is the positive counterpart
Of the negative sleeping experience
Of complete ignorance and absence of power.
Virat corresponds to the foot of the man
Standing on the bank of the river
And Visva to the reflected foot.
Visva is more consciously related to Virat
Than Taijasa to Hiranyagarbha
Or Prajna to Isvara,
As the foot is nearer to the reflected foot
Than the waist to the reflected waist
Or the head to the reflected head.
These illustrations show that
Waking is relatively more real
Than dream which has only a negative value.
The illustrations used here
Are to be taken in their spirit and not literally,
For, Visva, Taijasa and Prajna
Are not merely reflections
Of Virat, Hiranyagarbha and Isvara respectively,
But also their limitations
With qualities distorted
And experiences wrested from truth.

VI

As far as the manner of
Subjective experience is concerned,
It is true that what is within the mind
Is experienced as present in external objects.
But the objects themselves are not
Creations of the subjective mind.
There is a great difference between
Isvara-Srishti and Jiva-Srishti.
The existence of the objects
Belongs to Isvara-Srishti.
But the relation that exists between
The objects and the experiencing subject
Is Jiva-Srishti.
The Jiva is one of the contents of the Jagat
Which is Isvara-Srishti.
Hence, the Jiva cannot claim to be
The creator of the world,

Though it is the creator of
Its own subjective modes of
Psychological experience.
Waking experience is a perception.
Dream experience is a memory.
As perception precedes memory,
Waking precedes dream;
That is, dream is a remembrance
Of waking experiences
In the form of impressions.
To Brahman, the waking world is unreal.
But, to the individual or the Jiva
It is a relative fact
Lasting as long as
Individuality or Jivahood lasts.

VII

That the waking world has relative reality
Or Vyavaharika-Satta
Does not prove that it is real
In the absolute sense.
Comparatively waking is on a higher order
Than dream experiences,
For reasons already mentioned.
But, from the standpoint of the highest Reality,
Waking experience also is unreal.
As dream is transcended in the state of waking,
The world of waking too is transcended
In the state of Self-Realisation.

14. *Waking Experience is as False as Dream Experience*

Both in waking and in dream
Objects are "perceived" or "seen"
As different from the subject.
The character of "being seen"
Is common to both kinds of experience.
There is subject-object-relationship
In waking as well as in dream.
This is the similarity between the two.
"Something is seen as an object" means
"Something is other than the Self".
The experience of the not-self is illusory,
For, if the not-self were real,
The Self would be limited and unreal.
The illusory experience of the not-self
Is common to both waking and dream.
In waking, the mind experiences through the senses;
In dream, the mind alone experiences.
In both the states, the mind alone experiences
Whether externally or internally.
Dream is transcended by waking.
Waking is transcended by TURIYA.
Hence, both dream and waking are contradicted.
Waking contradicts dream,
And dream contradicts waking.
When the one is, the other is not.
Neither of the two is continuously existent,
This proves the unreality of both.

II

Duality is not real,
Because duality is the opposite of eternity.
Without duality there is no perception.
Hence, anything that is perceived is unreal
Whether in dream or in waking.
Dream is real when there is no waking.
Waking is real when there is no dream.
Hence, both are unreal experiences.
They depend on one another for their existence.
One cannot say whether he is dreaming or waking
Without referring one state to another state.
Desires are the rulers of all experiences
In waking and also in dream.
Waking is physical functioning of desires,

Dream is mental functioning of desires.
The senses are moved by desires in waking.
The mind is moved by desires in dreaming.
Both the states are like flowing streams.
They do not persist forever in one state.
That which persists forever is real.
Dream and waking have a beginning and an end.
Change is the character of all perceived objects.
Change implies non-existence at the beginning
And also at the end.
That which does not exist at the beginning
And does not exist at the end
Does not exist in the middle also.
Therefore waking is unreal like dream.

III

It may be objected by some that
Waking is real, because it is the cause of dream,
And dream is not the cause of waking.
But this objection is without support.
If waking is a cause,
It must be real.
If it is real,
It must exist forever.
Waking itself is without reality,
For it does not exist always.
If the cause itself is unreal,
How can it produce a real effect?
Both these are unreal states.
One who eats bellyful in waking state
May feel hungry in the dream state
And vice versa.
Things appear to be real only
In a particular condition.
They are not real always,
That which is not always real
Is an appearance and so unreal.

IV

Anything that has got a form
Is unreal.
Forms are special modes of cognition and perception.
They are not ultimate.
In waking there are physical forms.

In dreaming there are mental forms.
Anyhow all are forms only
Limited in space and time.
A form lasts only so long
As that particular mental condition lasts;
When there is a different mental condition
The forms of experience also change.
This is why the form of the world vanishes
When Self-Realisation is attained.

V

Both in dreaming and waking
External perceptions are considered as real
And internal functions as unreal (i.e., they are ignored).
If in waking we make a distinction
Between real and unreal,
In dream also we do the same thing.
Dream is real as long as it lasts,
Waking also is real as long as it lasts.
Dream is unreal from the standpoint of waking,
And equally so is waking to the dreamer.
From the standpoint of the highest Truth,
Waking is as false as dream.

VI

It may be said that objects in waking state
Serve some definite purpose
And those of dream do not serve a purpose.
This argument is incorrect
Because, the nature of serving a purpose
Which is seen in objects of waking
Is contradicted by dream and vice versa.
The utility and objective worth
Of Things, states, etc. in waking
Are cancelled in the dream state,
Even as the conditions and experiences in dream
Are invalidated in waking.
Objects act as means to ends
Only in a particular condition
And not in all conditions.
The causal relationship of waking
Is rendered nugatory in dream, and vice versa.
The logical sequence of waking
Is valid to itself alone and not to dreaming.

So is dream valid to its own state.
Waking and dreaming have their own notions of propriety,
And each is stultified by the other,
Though each appears to be real to itself.
Thus, the validity of both the states
Is rejected.

VII

It may be contended that
Objects of dream are queer, fantastic and unnatural,
And, hence, waking cannot be like dream.
But the experiences in dream
However grotesque or abnormal,
Are not abnormal to the dreamer.
They appear fantastic only in
A different state, viz. waking.
One cannot say what is really fantastic
And what is normal and real.
The mind gives values to objects
And its conception of normality and abnormality
Changes according to the state in which it is.
There is no permanent standard
Of normality, beauty or decorum,
Either in waking or in dreaming,
Which may hold good for all times.
The dreamer has his own conception
Of space, time and causation,
Even as the waking one has his own notions.
One state is absurd when compared to the other.
This shows that both states are illogical
And, therefore, absurd from the highest standpoint.

VIII

The world of waking experience is unreal,
Because it is the imagination of the cosmic mind.
The fact that in Self-Realisation
There is absolute cessation of phenomenal experience
Shows that all phenomena are unreal.
External forms are the expressions
Of the internal Sankalpas or willing.
Therefore, external objects have no real value.
They appear to exist only
As long as the Sankalpas exist.
The senses externalise the internal ideas

And present them in the forms of objects.
When the Sankalpas are drawn within
The world of objective experience vanishes in toto.
The Infinite Subject, viz., the Self alone remains.
There is no such thing as
Externality and internality in reality.
The ego and the non-ego,
The subject as well as the object,
All are imaginations of the mind alone.

IX

It may be said that
Objects seen in waking are not
Mere mental imaginations,
Because the objects of waking experience
Are seen by other people also,
Whether or not one's mind cognises them.
But it is seen that
In the dream state also
Objects of experience are open to
The perception of other people,
Though the people as well as the objects
Are all subjective imaginations.
It may be said that in waking
We perceive through the sense-organs
And not merely through ideas.
But it is seen that in dream also
We perceive through the sense-organs
Belonging to the dream-state,
Which are not less real than those of waking state.
As dream is unreal,
Waking also must be unreal.

X

The objective world of waking experience
Cannot have independent existence,
Because it is relative to the subject
Which cognises or perceives it.
The object is called an object
Just because there is a perceiving subject.
Similarly, a subject is called a subject
Just because there is a perceived object.
Neither of the two is self-existent,
And, therefore, both prove themselves to be unreal.

Subject and object appear
In the form of cause and effect.
Without a cause there is no effect,
Without an effect nothing can be a cause;
The conception of causation itself is illogical.
The mind perceives and recognises objects
Only by relating one thing to another.
The whole world of perception
Is a bundle of unintelligible relationships
Which the mind tries to organise into cause and effects.
Further, there is no causation at all,
Because, cause and effect are continuous.
There cannot be a lapse of time
In which the cause remains unchanged.
If the cause can exist unchanged for some time,
There is no reason why it should change at any time at all.
Either there is continuous causation,
Or no causation at all.
If causation is continuous,
Cause and effect become identical,
Being inseparable from one another.
If they are identical,
It means there is no causation at all.
If there is no causation,
There is no world of experience also.
The whole causal scheme is illogical,
Because it either requires the existence
Of a first uncaused cause,
Or it itself is meaningless.
There is no meaning in saying that
There is a first uncaused cause,
For, thereby, we create a beginning for time.
If causation were real,
It would never be possible to get rid of it.
But Self-Realisation breaks the chain of causation.
Hence, causation is false,
And, consequently, the world of experience
Also is false.
As in dream also there is experience
Of the causal series,
The waking world is false like the dream world.

15. Jagarat is as Unreal as Dream

For the Ajnanis or the worldly-minded persons the sensual objects are quite real. For the sages or those who are endowed with discrimination and enquiry they are unreal.

Whatever you see is false. There is no doubt in this. The deer sees water in the mirage when the sun is hot. They run towards the mirage for drinking water. They do not find any water there. The boy runs to take a piece of silver when there is bright sun. When he goes near the silver he does not find any silver. He finds only the mother-of-pearl. When a girl goes to bring water at night she sees a snake on her way and gets frightened. She takes a light to see the snake but finds only a rope. There is no snake there. A young man embraces a girl in his dream and experiences actual discharge of semen. When he wakes up he does not find a girl. You behold blueness in the sky. The sky appears as a blue dome. When one moves in the aeroplane in the sky he does not find any blue dome but the blue dome appears at a distance. Whatever you see do not really exist. They are mere illusory appearances like the objects in a dream. But the seer exists when the objects appear and disappear.

In the dream state big mountains, elephants, cities, big rivers etc. are seen within a minute Nadi called Hitanadi that is located in the throat. There is no space in the minute Nadi for these big things to remain there. Hence the dream objects are false or illusory. The objects that appear in the waking state also are false.

In the dream you witness the events of several years within a few minutes. Within a day of Brahma thousand Chaturyugas pass for us. Within the day of a Deva six months pass for us. Within the time taken by a huge mountain snake for a second meal, man takes his meals a hundred times. Within the time taken by a child to develop itself in the womb, small insects take time to generate crores of their progeny. A happy man spends one night like a minute whereas a man who is drowned in grief spends one night like several years. Hence time also does not appear to be the same at all times for all. The objects that appear and perish in time are illusory.

The thing seen by you in your dream is not seen in the same place and in the same manner in the waking state. In the same manner one may say that Mr. X is a good man. The same man appears as a bad man for another.

The objects seen in a dream do not exist correctly in the waking state. The objects seen in the waking state appear different even in the waking state also. In the dream state you do not recollect the things of the waking state. You do not recollect the things in the dreaming state, "I saw such and such objects in the waking state. I do not see them now." Therefore the objects of the waking state are more false than the objects of the dream. Srutis and sages declare that the objects of the world are as false as the objects of the dream. They call the world Deergha-Svapna or a long dream.

That which does not exist in the beginning and in the end does not really exist in the middle also. It is unreal. The snake that is found in the rope at night does not exist when a lamp is brought. It appears in the middle only. Such is the case with silver in the mother-of-pearl, water in the mirage, city in the clouds, etc. Therefore they are unreal even when they appear. The dream objects also do not exist in the daytime. Similarly the objects of this world appear in the middle only. Hence they are unreal.

An objector says: "The food and drink that you take in the waking state give you satisfaction. But hunger is not appeased by the food taken in dream. Therefore the objects of the dream are false. The objects of the waking state are true." A man who goes to sleep after taking a sumptuous meal in the waking state suffers from the pangs of hunger in the dream. He who enjoys a good feast in the dream becomes very hungry as soon as he wakes up. Similarly the results of actions done in the waking state are not seen in the dream and vice versa. Therefore, the waking state is as false as dream.

An objector says, "A man dreams that he has four hands and that he is flying in the air. Is this not false? Jagrat state is not like this. Therefore it is true." A man obtains the birth of a Deva or animal or a bird on account of his Karmas. He becomes Indra with thousand hands in the waking state. He becomes a bird and flies in the air in the waking state. He becomes animal with four legs, a centipede with hundred feet or a snake without feet. Therefore waking state and dream state are same. Just as in dream some objects are false, some are true, so also in waking state some objects like the snake in the rope are false, some like jar, cloth are true. The objects of the dream and waking state are not so absolutely true as Atman or Brahman.

Just as you remove a thorn by a thorn, just as you remove the dirt of the cloth by another dirt—the salt-earth, just as you cut the iron by another iron only, so also you will have to take recourse to another false object like a Guru or a God, though Atman or Brahman alone is everything. A false object in the dream produces real fear and wakes you up. Sometimes whatever you see in dream turns out to be true. An unreal woman in dream causes a real discharge of semen. Although God and Guru are not so real as Brahman, they are boats to help you to cross this Samsara or ocean of births and deaths. Without their grace you cannot attain immortality or eternal bliss.

Atma Svarup! Brahman alone is really existent. Jiva, world are false! Kill this illusory egoism. The world is unreal when compared to Brahman. It is a solid reality for a passionate worldly man, even as dreams are real to the childish. The world does not exist for a Jnani or a Mukta.

16. Remove The Colouring of The Mind

In days of yore there were very able dyers in Marwar or Rajputana. They would give seven colours to the sari or clothes of ladies. After washing the cloth one colour will fade away. Another colour will shine. After some washing a third colour will manifest in the cloth; then a fourth colour and so on. Even so the mind is coloured when it associates with the different objects of the world. When the mind is Sattvic, it has white colour; when it is Rajasic, it is tinged with red colour; when it is Tamasic it has a black colour.

The mind plays with the five senses of perception and gets experiences in the waking state. The impressions are lodged in the causal body or Karana Sarira. Ajnana or causal body is like a black sheet of cloth. In it are contained the Samskaras of all your previous births.

The mind is ever rotating like a wheel. It receives the different sense-impressions through the avenues of the senses.

In the dream state the doors or windows of the senses are shut. The mind remains alone and plays. It is the subject and it is the object. It projects various sorts of objects like mountains, rivers, gardens, chariots, cars, etc., from its own body from the material collected during the waking state. It manufactures curious mixtures and marvellous combinations. Sometimes the experiences of the previous births that are lodged in the causal body flash out during the dreaming state.

Remove the colouring of the mind through meditation on Atman. Do not allow the mind to run into the sensual grooves. Fortify yourself by developing the Vijnanamaya Kosha or intellect through Vichara or enquiry of Brahman, reflection and contemplation. The Vijnanamaya Kosha will serve the purpose of a strong fortress. It will not allow the sense-impressions to be lodged in the causal body. It will not allow the impressions of the causal body to come out. It will serve a double purpose.

You will be free from dreams through meditation on the Supreme Being or Brahman when the colouring of the mind has been removed.

Brahma Jnanis or Sages have no dreams.

May you all attain the Turiya or the fourth state of eternal bliss, which transcends the three states of waking, dream and deep sleep!

17. *Upanishads And Dreams*

"The Purusha has only two abodes, this and the next world. The dream state, which is the third is at the junction of the two. Abiding at the junction he sees the two abodes, this and the next world. In proportion the endeavour with which one is striving to obtain the place of the other world does he accordingly see both suffering and bliss. When he dreams he takes away a little of the impressions of this world which consists of all elements (the waking state), himself puts the body aside and himself creates a dream body in its place, revealing his own splendour by his own light and dreams. In this state the Purusha himself becomes unmingled light." (Bri. Up. IV.iii.9.)

"There are no chariots, nor horses to be yoked to them, nor roads there, but he creates the chariots, horses and the roads. There are no pleasures, joys or delights, but he creates the pleasures, joys and delights. There are no tanks, no lakes or rivers there, but he creates the tanks, lakes and rivers, for he is the agent." (Ibid. IV.iii.10.)

"The God-like Purusha who moves alone puts the body aside in the dream state and himself awake and taking the shining functions of the organs with him, watches those that are asleep. Again he comes to the waking state." (Ibid. IV.iii.11.)

"The radiant Purusha who is immortal and moves alone, preserves the unclean rest of the body by the power of the vital force and roams out of the rest. Himself immortal, he proceeds where his desire leads him." (Ibid. IV.iii.12.)

"In the dream world, the shining one attains higher and lower states and assumes manifold forms. He seems to be enjoying himself in the company of women or laughing or beholding fearful sights." (Ibid. IV.iii.13.)

"Everybody sees his sport but nobody sees him." They say, "Do not wake him up suddenly". If the Purusha does not return to the waking state through the same doors of the senses through which he entered into the state of dream, if he re-enters in any other manner, then diseases are produced such as blindness, deafness etc. which are difficult to be cured. Some day indeed that the dream state of a man is the same as his waking state as he sees in dreams only those things that he sees in the waking state. This is not so because in the dream state the Purusha becomes a self-shining light." (Ibid. IV.iii.14.)

"After enjoying himself and roaming and merely seeing the results of the good and evil in dreams, he rests in a state of deep sleep. He comes back in a reverse order to his former condition, the dream state. He is not touched by whatever he beholds in that state, because the Purusha is unattached." (Ibid. IV.iii.15.)

"After enjoying himself and wandering in the waking state and after seeing what is holy and sinful, the results of good and evil, he proceeds again in the reverse order to his former condition, the dream state or the deep sleep." (Ibid. IV.iii.17.)

"Just as a large fish swims alternately to both the banks of the river, the right and the left one or the Eastern and Western, so the Purusha glides between both boundaries—the boundary of dream and the boundary of the waking state." (Ibid. IV.iii.18.)

"In him are those Nadis called Hita, which are as fine as a hair split into a thousand parts, and filled with white, blue, yellow, green and red juice.

"Therefore all the objects of terror, which a man sees when awake, are ignorance fancied by him in dream, when anybody seems to kill him, sees to overpower him, an elephant seems to put him to fight when he falls into a pit. Again when he seems to be conscious, "I am God. I am King. I am even all this," he has attained the highest peace.

"When the individual soul is in the state of dream, he becomes an Emperor as it were or a noble Brahmana as it were, or attains states high or low, as it were. Just as an Emperor, taking his followers, moves about as he pleases, so does the soul, taking the organs move about as he pleases in his own body. (Ibid. II.i.18.)

"Because in dream the dreamer does not actually do what is holy or evil; he is not chained by either; for good or evil actions and their consequences are not imputed to the mere spectator for them.

"Having in that dream enjoyed pleasure, wandered about and seen what is holy and sinful, he proceeds again in the reverse order to the place of birth, to the waking state. He is not chained by what he sees there, for, Purusha is untouched." (Ibid. IV.3.16.)

18. *Prasna-Upanishad on Dreams*

(Prasna Up. IV-1 to 9)

Then Gargya the grandson of Surya questioned Pippalada:

"O Bhagavan! What are they that sleep in man? What wake in him? Which is the Deva who sees dreams? Whose is this bliss? On what do all these depend?"

Pippalada replied: O Gargya! Just as the rays of the sun, when setting, become one in that disc of light and come forth again when the sun rises again, so all of these become one in the highest Deva—the mind. Therefore, at that time, that man does not hear, see, smell, taste, feel, does not speak, nor take, nor enjoy, nor evacuate, nor move; they say 'he sleeps'.

The fires of Prana alone are awake in the city (body). The Apana is the Garhapatya fire. Vyana is the Anvaharya-pachana fire. The Prana is the Ahavaniya fire, because it is taken out of Garhapatya fire.

Because the Samana distributes equally the oblations, the inspiration and expiration, he is the priest (Hotri). The mind is the sacrifice, the Udana is the reward of the sacrifice; he leads the sacrifices every day (in deep sleep to Brahman).

In this state, this Deva (mind) enjoys in dream his greatness. What has been seen, he sees again, what has been heard, he hears again, what has been enjoyed in different countries and quarters, he enjoys again. What has been seen and not seen, heard and not heard, experienced and not experienced, real and unreal, he sees all; he being all, sees.

When he is overpowered by light, then that God (mind) sees no dreams and at that time the bliss arises in this body.

Just as, O beloved one, birds repair to a tree to roost (dwell), so indeed all this rests in the Supreme Atman.

The earth and the subtle elements, the water and its subtle elements, the fire and its subtle elements, the air and its subtle elements, Akasa and its subtle elements, the eye and what can be seen, the ear and what can be heard, the nose and what can be smelt, taste and what can be tasted, touch and its objects, speech and its objects, the hands and what can be grasped, the feet and what can be walked, the organ of generation and what is to be enjoyed, the organ of excretion and what must be excreted, the mind and what must be thought of, the intellect and what must be determined, egoism and its object, Chitta and its object, light and its object, Prana and what is to be supported by it—(all these rest in the Supreme Atman in deep sleep.)

It is he who sees, feels, hears, smells, tastes, thinks, knows; he is the doer, the intelligent soul, the Purusha. He dwells in the highest, indestructible Self.

19. Dream

(From Mandukyopanishad—4)

The second quarter is the Taijasa whose sphere or field or place is dream, who is conscious of internal objects, who has seven limbs and nineteen mouths and who enjoys the subtle objects.

During dream, the mind creates various kinds of objects out of the impressions produced by the experiences of the waking state. The mind reproduces the whole of its waking life in dream through the force of Avidya (ignorance), Kama (desire or imagination) and Karma (action). The mind is the perceiver and the mind itself is the perceived in the dream. The mind creates the objects without the help of any external means. It creates various curious, fantastic mixtures. You may witness in the dream that your living father is dead, that you are flying in the air. You may see in the dream a lion with the head of an elephant, a cow with the head of a dog. The desires that are not satisfied during the waking state are gratified in the dream. Dream is a mysterious phenomenon. It is more interesting than the waking state.

Svapna or dream is that state during which Atman (Taijasa) experiences through the mind associated with the Vasanas of the waking condition, sound and other objects which are of the form of the Vasanas created for the time being, even in the absence of the gross sound and the others. Like a businessman tired of worldly acts, in the waking state the individual soul strives to find the path to retire into his abode within. The Svapna Avastha is that in which when the senses are at rest, there is the manifestation of the knower and the known along with the affinities (Vasanas) of things enjoyed in the waking state. In this state Visva alone, his actions in the waking state having ceased, reaches the state of Taijasa (of Tejas, effulgence or essence of light), who moves in the middle of the Nadis (nerves), illuminates by his lustre, the heterogeneity of the subtle dream world which is the form of Vasanas (affinities), and himself enjoys according to his wish.

Sutratman or Hiranyagarbha, under the orders of Isvara, having entered the microcosmic subtle body and having Manas (mind) as his vehicle, reaches the Taijasa state. Then he goes by the names of Taijasa, Pratibhasika and Svapnakalpita (the one bred out of dream).

The dreamer creates the world of his own in the dreaming state. Mind alone works independently in this state. The senses are withdrawn into the mind. The senses are at rest. Just as a man withdraws himself from the outside world, closes the door and windows of his room and works within the room, so also the mind withdraws itself from the outside world and plays in the dream world with the Vasanas and Samskaras and enjoys objects made up of fine or subtle ideas which are the products of desire. Dream is a mere play of the mind only. The mind itself projects all sorts of subtle objects from its own body through the potentiality of impressions of the waking state (Vasanas) and enjoys these objects. Therefore there is a very subtle experience by Taijasa in the form of Vasanas only, whereas the experience of the waking state by Visva is gross.

You will find in Brihadaranyaka Upanishad IV-iii-9, "He sleeps full of the impressions produced by the varied experience of the waking state and experiences dreams. He takes with him the impressions of the world during the waking state, destroys and builds them up again and experiences dream by his own light." The Atharvana-veda says, "All these are in the mind. They are experienced or cognised by the Taijasa." The experiencer of the dream state is called Taijasa, because he is entirely of the essence of light.

Just as pictures are painted on the canvas, so also the impressions of the waking state are painted in the canvas-mind. The pictures on the canvas seem to possess various dimensions though it is on a plane surface only. Even so, though the dream-experiences are really states of the mind only, the experiencer experiences internality and externality in the dream world. He feels while dreaming that the dream world is quite real.

Pravivikta: Pra—differentiated; vivikta—from the objects of the state. The objects perceived in the waking state have an external reality common to all beings, whereas the objects perceived in the dreams are revivals of impressions received in the waking state and have an external reality only to the dreamer.

Antahprajna: Inward consciousness; the experiencer is conscious of the dream world only. Pravivikta or subtle is that which manifests itself in dreams, being impressions of objects perceived in the waking state. The state of consciousness by which these subtle objects are perceived is called Antahprajna or inner perception. The impressions of the waking state remain in the mind, which independent of the senses are perceived in the dream. The mind is more internal than the senses. The dreamer is conscious of the mental states which are the impressions left in the mind by the previous Jagrat Avastha or waking state. Hence it is called Antah-prajna.

The microcosmic aspect of Atman in the subtle or mental state is called Taijasa and His macrocosmic aspect is known as Hiranyagarbha. Just as Virat is one with Visva in the waking state, so also Taijasa is one with Hiranyagarbha in the dreaming state.

20. The Story of a Dreamer Subhoda

Subodha was born in a Brahmin family in the ancient capital of Indraprastha. He was leading a pure life. He was second to none in learning. He was piety and compassion incarnate. He had every virtue that could be desired. He was highly charitable and God-minded. He was a Godly personality. He was God living on earth. He was a perfect celibate.

One fine day Subhoda took a refreshing bath, had a sumptuous meal. It was midday on a midsummer. It was terribly sultry. He felt exhausted and leaned against a low couch. He felt drowsy and fell into the state of dream. In his dream he became the son of the King of Kasi. He grew up to the age of 12. His father, the king of Kasi educated him in all the Vidyas suitable to a Prince. The prince was named Priyadarshi. Prince Priyadarshi soon picked up all the arts, archery etc. The king of Kasi prepared the marriage of his son in proper time. Prince Priyadarshi was installed on the throne and the king retired. Priyadarshi ruled the country justly and wisely.

One day King Priyadarshi went on a hunting expedition with a retinue of followers. He had a very good game. He was extremely tired. His retinue had fallen back. He was far away from them. He tied the horse to a tree. He went to a hut and demanded water for drinking. A beautiful lady equal in beauty to a celestial damsel brought a glassful of water. The king was enchanted by the beauty of the lady. He wanted to marry her. The father of the woman also agreed on condition that he remained with them and gave half of his wealth in return. The king agreed.

The king took the newly wedded wife to the kingdom. She turned to be a wretched woman. She ill-treated every one. She led the king into all evil ways which the king was not at all habituated to. He led a very loose life. He became very unpopular in the country. He was disliked by all because he never cared for the welfare of the people. All the day and night he was engaged in the company of the wicked new queen. He had many sons and daughters by his new wife. He led a despicable life in her company.

One night King Priyadarshi retired to his bedchamber after a long day of dissipation and sensuous revelling. He laid himself upon the bed soon and sank into a sound slumber. King Priyadarshi dreamt that his death took place and people were carrying his dead body. He then found himself reborn in the house of a Bania. The Bania was a wine seller. He too took the profession and led the life of a wine seller throughout his life. One day he drank plenty of wine. He fell into drunkard stupor. In that condition he dreamt that he was born as a Sudra in the country of Usinara. He served the King of Usinara as a stable keeper. The whole life he was tending the horses. One night he dreamt that he was born as Chandala and was leading the life as such. One day he went to the forest to collect fuel. He was attacked by a tiger. He shrieked and woke up to find himself to be once again Subhoda, the Brahmin leaning on his couch.

Subhoda clearly and vividly perceived his various lives as King Priyadarshi, as the son of a Bania, as a Sudra and as a Chandala. He lived several lives. All these he experienced in one single dream.

O Man! You are like Subhoda. Just as Subhoda shrieked when the tiger attacked him you are also now under the painful agony of your present life. You find everywhere selfishness, crookedness, wars and calamities. There is no food to eat. There is no peace of mind. You are entangled in the meshes of Maya and Tamas. You are lazy and lethargic. You are sometimes fed up with life. Sometimes you even want to commit suicide when you are placed in acute suffering in your private and public life. You find your ambitions are shattered. You fall in evil company. You spoil your life and youth. You have endless desires.

Friend, tell me frankly: "How long you want to remain in this state of abject ignorance and suffering"? Wake up. Gird up your loins. Become a Yogi. You are not this physical body. You have nothing to do with suffering. Shake of this lethargy. Open your eyes. Enough of your long slumber. Wake up! Wake up to the Reality! Now it is Brahmamuhurtha, the dawn of glorious future! Sleep no more. Identify yourself with the real spirit within. You will no more be tormented by agony and misery.

Rise up in the ladder of Yoga. Follow the instructions of the ancient seers and sages. Practise Namasmarana. Give up vanity. Be humble and simple. Lead a life of purity, goodness and nobility. You will shine as a dynamic Yogi!

May you bring light, joy and peace to the Whole world! May you become Immortal!

21. Raja Janaka's Dream

Raja Janaka ruled over the country of Videha. He was once reclining on a sofa. It was the middle of the day in the hot month of June. He had a short nap for a few seconds. He dreamt that a rival king with a large army had invaded his country and slew his soldiers and ministers. He was driven out of his palace barefooted and without any clothes covering him.

Janaka found himself roaming about in a jungle. He was thirsty and hungry. He reached a small town where he begged for food. No one paid any attention to his entreaties. He reached a place where some people were distributing food to the beggars. Each beggar had an earthen bowl to receive rice water. Janaka had no bowl and so they turned him out to bring a bowl. He went in search of a vessel. He requested other beggars to lend him a bowl, but none would part with his bowl. At last Janaka found a broken piece of a bowl. Now he ran to the spot where rice water was distributed. All the foodstuff had been already distributed.

Raja Janaka was very much tired on account of long travelling, hunger and thirst and heat of the summer. He stretched himself near a fireplace where foodstuff was cooked. Here some one took pity over Janaka. He gave him some rice water which was found at the bottom of a vessel. Janaka took it with intense joy and just as he put it to his lips, two large bulls tumbled fighting over him. The bowl was broken to pieces. The Raja woke up with great fear.

Janaka was trembling violently. He was in a great dilemma as to which of his two states was real. All the time he was in dream, he never thought that it was an illusion and that the misery of hunger and thirst and his other troubles were unreal.

The queen asked Janaka, "O Lord! What is the matter with you?" The only words which Janaka spoke were, "Which is real, this or that?" From that time he left all his work and became silent. He uttered nothing but the above words.

The ministers thought that Janaka was suffering from some disease. It was announced by them that anyone who cured the Raja will be richly rewarded and those who fail to cure the Raja will be made life prisoners. Great physicians and specialists began to pour in and tried their luck, but no one could answer the query of the Raja. Hundreds of Brahmins well versed in the science of curing diseases were put in the state prison.

Among the prisoners was also the father of the great sage Ashtavakra. When Ashtavakra was a boy of only ten years of age, he was told by his mother that his father was a state prisoner because he failed to cure Raja Janaka. He at once started to see Janaka. He asked the Raja if he desired to hear the solution of his questions in a brief and few words as the question itself is put or full details of his dream experience may be recited. Janaka did not like to have his humiliating dream repeated in presence of a big gathering. He consented to receive a brief answer.

Ashtavakra then whispered into the ear of Janaka, "Neither this nor that is real." Raja Janaka at once became joyful. His confusion was removed.

Raja Janaka then asked Ashtavakra, "What is real?" There upon there was a long dialogue between him and the sage. This is recorded in the well-known book, "Ashtavakra Gita," which is highly useful for all seekers after Truth.

22. Goudapadacharya on Dreams

Men of knowledge have declared the unreality of everything that is seen in the dream, because all these objects of the dream are located within the body and exist in a confined space.

All these entities like mountains, elephants etc., are seen in the dream only inside the body. Therefore, they cannot be real.

And on account of the shortness of the time, it is impossible for the dreamer to go out of the body and perceive the objects of dream. And when the dreamer wakes up, he does not find himself in the place even in the dream. It is not a fact that all that is seen in the dream can be situated in a limited space. And a man sleeping in the east, very often feels himself as it were, experiencing dreams in the north. As soon as a man falls asleep he begins to dream objects, as it were, at a place hundreds of miles away from his body, which he can reach only after a month or so in the waking state. His going to such a long distance and coming back to his body within half a day (one night) is not a fact. Hence this is unreal that he goes out of the body. He dreams of some place but he wakes up in another place where he slept the previous day.

Though a man goes to sleep at night he feels as if he is seeing objects in the daytime and meeting many persons in the broad daylight. But this meeting is found to be false. Therefore the dream is a falsity.

The Sruti declares the illustration of the state of dream, by saying, "there are no chariots" etc. This assertion is based on reason.

Moreover the different objects perceived in the dream are unreal even though they are perceived to exist. For the same reason the objects of the waking state are illusory. The nature of the objects is not different in the waking and the dreaming states. The only difference is in the limitation of space connected with the object. The fact of being seen is commonly illusory in both states.

Further, the waking and dreaming states are same since the objects perceived in both states are same. That which is non-existent at the beginning and also non-existent in the end, is necessarily non-existent in the middle. The objects we see are thus only illusions, though we regard them as real, due to our ignorance of the Reality of the Atman.

The objects used as means to some and or purpose in the waking state are contradicted in the dream state. A man in the waking state, eats and drinks and appeases his hunger and is free from thirst. But when he goes to sleep, he finds himself in dream again afflicted with hunger and thirst as if he has not taken food and drink for days together. And the contrary also happens and is found to be true. A person who has taken full meal and drink in the dream finds himself afflicted with hunger and thirst as soon as he wakes up from sleep. Hence we establish the illusoriness of the objects of both the waking and the dreaming states.

The objects perceived in dream are all usually, met with in the waking state, and those which are not met with in the waking state own their existence to the peculiar conditions or circumstances in which his mind is working for the time being. Just as Indra, etc., who reside in heaven have thousand eyes, etc., on account of their existence in heaven, so also there are the abnormal peculiar features of the dreamer due to the peculiar conditions of the state of dream. All these objects are but the imaginations of his own mind. It is just like the case of a person in the waking state, who, while going to another country sees on the way objects belonging to the place. Just as snake in the rope and mirage in the desert are unreal and are mere mental imaginations, so are the objects of dream and waking experience.

In the dream state also those which are mere modifications of the mind cognised within are illusory. For, those internal objects vanish the moment they are perceived. Objects perceived outside are considered as real. Similarly in the waking state objects known as real and mental imaginations should be considered as unreal. Objects, both external and internal, are mere creations of the mind whether it is in the dream or in the waking state.

23. Sri Nimbarkacharya on Dreams

As some dreams are indicative of future good or bad fortunes, it is impossible for the individual to dream a good or a bad dream according to his own choice, he, being in his present state of bondage, ignorant of the future. The individual soul, in his emancipated state, can certainly exercise his will for the creation of vision in dreams; but the power, in the state of his bondage, remains eclipsed by the superior will of the Universal Soul, who directs his actions according to the merits and demerits of his past conduct; and the suppression of his power is due to his being encaged in the body.

The creation in dream is all the doing of the Universal soul; as it is of a strange and illusive character, being not entirely true, nor entirely untrue; and as such, it cannot be done by the individual soul, for his essential characteristics including creative powers, in the present state of bondage, are as yet unrealised; as he is limited and conditioned, his inherent powers cannot have full play; and therefore it is not possible for him to create the strange things of dream.

So the Universal Soul is the creator of dreams and not the individual soul; for had it been possible for him to shape his dreams, he would never have dreamt a bad dream, but would always have dreamt only propitious ones.

24. Dream of Chuang Tze

Chuang Tze, a Chinese Philosopher, once dreamt that he was a butterfly. On waking, he said to himself, "Now, am I a man dreaming that I am a butterfly, or am I a butterfly thinking that I am a man?"

One night when Chuang Tze lay in bed,
He dreamed he was a butterfly,
Then waking himself he said,
To solve this problem now I'll try;
Am I a man I've wondered long,
Or butterfly that thinks I'm Chuang?

25. Dream Hints

I

Dreams and Death are rock foundations of all philosophy. Dream world is totally different from the waking world. But some facts are strikingly common to both. (1) Sometimes we have a dream within a dream. (2) During sleep, sometimes we are conscious of the fact that we are asleep and we are dreaming. (3) In dreams more often than not we assume a body that is the master of the dream world. (4) Sometimes we feel extremely helpless amidst the facts of the dream world. We cry and we weep to the extent that the physiological system is affected. From these facts of common experience some conclusions can be drawn. It will be readily conceded: (a) that cognitive, connotive and affective processes are as much owned by dream personality as by the personality of the waking subjects; (b) that in the handling of the facts of the dream world, reason operates subject to the laws of the dream world in the same manner as it operates in the physical world subject to the laws of physics. Since the law of the two worlds widely differ, the fruits of the operations of reason must be necessarily different, e.g., Reason helps the man to cross the ocean in the dream by bodily flight in the air; it can never suggest the same thing in the physical world. Such a suggestion would belong to the realm of imagination in the waking world; (c) that Introspection brings even to the dream personality (d) that there is some sort of interaction between the dream personality and the psychological waking self that in its turn affects that physiological system and finally (e) in connection with the foregoing interaction, it must be noted that it is the mind-stuff that makes interaction possible. The facts of the two worlds although very much similar have no line of continuity except through the medium of the mind stuff. Thus however much we may know about the facts of the different worlds, there must remain discontinuity between the two worlds and unless we have discovered the common continuum i.e. the mind stuff.

II

When you dream you see the events of fifty years within an hour. You actually feel that fifty years have passed. Which is correct, the time of one hour of waking consciousness or the fifty years of dreaming consciousness? Both are correct. The waking state and the dreaming state are of the same quality of nature. They are equal (Samana). The only difference is that the waking state is a long dream or Deergha Svapna.

In dream the Samskaras of your previous births, which are imbedded in your Karana Sarira (causal body), will assume forms and become dream picture.

III

The difference between the waking and the dreaming states consists in this, that in the waking condition the mind depends on the outwards impressions, while in the dreaming state it creates its impressions and enjoys them. It uses, of course, the materials of the waking state. Jagrat is a long dream state only (Deergha Svapna).

Manorajya (building castles in the air), recollection of the events and things of dream, recollection of things long past in the waking state all are Svapna Jagrat (Dreaming in the waking state).

When the mind enters the Hita Nadi which proceeds from the heart and surrounds the great membrane round the heart, which is as thin as a hair divided into thousand parts and is filled with the minute essence of various colours of white, black, yellow and red, the individual soul or Jiva (ego) experiences the state of dream (Svapna Avastha).

You dream that you are a king. You enjoy various kinds of royal pleasures. As soon as you wake up, everything vanishes. But you do not feel for the loss because you know that the dream creatures are all false. Even in the waking consciousness if you are well established in the idea that the world is a false illusion, you will not get any pain.

When you know the real Tattva (Brahman) the waking consciousness also will become quite false like a dream. Wake up and realise! my child.

There is temperamental difference. Some rarely get dreams. A Jnani who has knowledge of the Self will have no dreams.

During dream you see splendid, effulgent light. Where does it come from? From Atman. The light that is present in the dream clearly indicates that Atman is self-luminous (Svayam Jyoti, Sva Prakasa).

When modified by the impressions which the external objects have left, it (the Jiva) sees dreams.

In dream state the senses are quiet and absorbed in the mind. The mind alone operates in a free and unfettered manner. The mind itself assumes the various forms of bee, flower, mountain, elephant, horse, river etc. The seer and the seen are one.

26. Dream-Symbols And Their Meanings

Abuse: There may be a dispute between you and the person with whom you do business. Take heed and be not slack in your attentions.

Accident: Personal afflictions may be inevitable. But you will remove soon from the trouble.

Accuse: This is a sign of great trouble. You will acquire riches by your own personal efforts.

Adultery: Troubles are approaching. Your prospects may be blasted. Despair will catch hold of you.

Advancement: A sign of success in all that you undertake.

Advocate: A dream that you are an advocate indicates that you will be prominent in future. You will win universal respect.

Affluence: This is not a favourable dream. It is indicatory of poverty.

Anger: The person with whom you are angry is your best friend.

Ass: All your great troubles, in spite of despairing circumstances, will end in ultimate success after much struggle and suffering.

Baby: If you are nursing a baby, it denotes sorrow and misfortune. If you see a baby that is sick, it means that somebody among your relatives will die.

Bachelor: Dreaming of a bachelor tells that you will shortly, meet with a friend.

Bankrupt: This is a dream of warning lest you should undertake something undesirable for you and also injurious to yourself. Be cautious in your transactions.

Battle: To dream of being in a battle means quarrel with neighbours or friends in a serious manner.

Beauty: To dream that you are beautiful indicates that you will become ugly with sickness and that you will become weak in body. Increasing beauty indicates death.

Birds: To see birds flying are very unlucky; it denotes sorrowful setback in circumstances. Poor persons may become better especially if they hear birds sing.

Birth: For unmarried women to dream of giving of birth to children, is indicative of inevitable unchastity. For married women it indicates happy confinement.

Blind: To dream of the blind is a sign that you will have no real friends.

Boat: To sail in a boat or ship on smooth waters is lucky. On rough waters, it is unlucky. To fall into water indicates great peril.

Books: To dream of books is an auspicious sign. Your future life will be very agreeable. Woman dreaming of books will get a son of eminent learning.

Bread: You will succeed in earthly business pursuits. Eating good bread indicates good health and long life. Burnt bread is a sign of funeral and so is bad.

Bride, Bridegroom: This dream is an unlucky one. It indicates sorrow and disappointment. You will mourn at the death of some relative.

Bugs: This indicates sure sickness. Many enemies are seeking to injure you.

Butter: Good dream. Joy and feasting. Sufferings terminate quickly.

Camel: Heavy burdens will come upon you. You will meet with heavy disasters. But you will bear with heroism.

Cat: This is a bad dream. This indicates treachery and fraud. Killing a cat indicates discovery of enemies.

Cattle: You will become rich and fortunate. Black and big-horned cattle indicate enemies of a violent nature.

Children: See Birth.

Clouds: Dark clouds indicate great sorrows that have to be passed through. But they will pass away if the clouds are moving or breaking away.

Corpse: Vision of a corpse indicates a hasty and imprudent engagement in which you will be unhappy.

Cow: Milking cow is a sign of riches. To be pursued by a cow indicates an overtaking enemy.

Crow: This indicates a sorrowful funeral ceremony.

Death: This indicates long life. But a sick person dreaming of death has the positive results.

Desert: Travelling across a desert shows the inevitability of a long and tedious journey. Accompaniment of sunshine indicates successful journey.

Devil: It is high time for you to mend yourself. Great evil may come to you. You must pursue virtue.

Dinner: If you are taking your dinner, it foretells great difficulties where you will be in want of meals. You will be uncomfortable. Enemies will try to injure your character. You should be careful about those whom you are confiding.

Disease: If a sick person dreams of disease it means recovery from the same. To young men it is a warning against evil company and intemperance.

Earthquake: This foretells that great trouble is going to come, loss in business, bereavement and separation. Family ties are broken by death—quarrels in family and fear everywhere, heart breaking agony and disaster from all sides.

Eclipse: Hopes are eclipsed. Death is near. Enjoyment may be put an end to. There is no use of dotting on the wife, for life is coming to an end. The friend is a traitor. All expectations will bear no fruit.

Elephant: Good health, success, strength, prosperity, intelligence.

Embroidery: Those persons who love you are not true to their salt. They will deceive you.

Famine: National prosperity and individual comfort. Much enjoyment. A dream of contrary.

Father: Father loves you. If the father is dead, it shows a sign of affliction.

Fields: Very great prosperity. To walk in green fields shows great happiness and wealth. Everything happens good. Scorched fields denote poverty.

Fighting: Quarrels in families. Misunderstanding among lovers, if not temporary separation. A bad dream for merchants, soldiers and sailors.

Fire: Health and great happiness, kind relations and warm friends.

Floods: Successful trade, safe voyage for traders. But to ordinary persons it indicates bad health and unfavourable circumstances.

Flowers: Gathering beautiful flowers is an indication of prosperity. You will be very fortunate in all your undertakings.

Frogs: These creatures are not harmful. This dream therefore is not unfavourable. It denotes success.

Ghost: This is a very bad omen. Difficulties will be overwhelming. Terrible enemies will overpower you.

Giant: Great difficulty to be encountered. But meet it with boldness. Then it will vanish. This indicates that you will have an enemy of the most dreadful character.

Girl (unmarried): Success, auspiciousness will come over you. Hopes will be fulfilled.

God: This is a rare dream which few people experience. Great success and elevation.

Grave: Some friend or relative will die. Recovery from illness doubtful.

Hanging: If you are hung, it is good to you. You will rise in society, and become wealthy.

Heaven: The remainder of your life will be spiritually happy, and your death will be peaceful.

Hell: There will be bodily suffering and also mental agony. Great suffering due to enemies and death of relatives, etc.

Home: To dream of home-life in early boyhood indicates good health and prosperity. Good sign of progress.

Husband: Your wish will not be granted. If you fall in love with another woman's husband, it indicates that you are growing vicious.

Ill: To dream that you are ill shows that you will have to fall a victim to some temptation, which, if you do not resist, will injure your character.

Injury: If you are injured by somebody else, it means that there are enemies to destroy you. Beware of them. Change of locality is desirable.

Itch: This is an unlucky dream. Denotes much difficulty and trouble. You will be unhappy.

Jail: If you dream that you are in jail it indicates that in life you will prosper. This is a dream of contrary.

Journey: This indicates that there will be a great change in conditions and circumstances. Good journey indicates good conditions and bad journey with troubles indicates a bad life.

King: To appear before a friendly king is a sign of great success, and before a cruel king is very unfavourable.

Lamp: Very favourable dream. Very happy life. Family peaceful. This dream is always of good signs.

Learning: You will attain influence and respect. Good omen to dream that you are learning and acquiring knowledge.

Leprosy: To dream that you have leprosy always indicates a very great future misfortune. Perhaps you have committed some crime to be severely punished by law. You will have many enemies.

Light: To dream of lights is very good. It denotes riches and honour.

Limbs: Breakage of limbs indicates breakage of a marriage vow.

Lion: This dream indicates greatness, elevation and honour. You will become very important among men. You will become very powerful and happy.

Money: Receiving money in dream denotes earthly prosperity. Giving of it denotes ability to give money.

Mother: If you dream that you see your mother and converse with her, it indicates that you will have prosperity in life. To dream that you have lost your mother indicates her sickness.

Murder: To dream that you have murdered somebody denotes that you are going to become very bad and wretched, vicious and criminal.

Nectar: To drink nectar in dream indicates riches and prosperity. You will be beyond your expectations. You will marry a handsome person in high life and live in great state.

Nightmare: You are guided by foolish persons. Beware of such people.

Noises: To dream of hearing noises indicates quarrels in family and much misery in life.

Ocean: The state of life will be as the ocean is perceived to be in dream, viz., calm and peaceful life when the ocean is calm and troublesome life when the ocean is stormy, etc.

Office: If you dream that you are turned out of the office it means that you will die or lose all property. This is a very bad dream for all people.

Owl: Denotes sickness and poverty, disgrace and sorrow. After dreaming of an owl, one need not have any hope of prosperity in life.

Palace: To live in a palace is a good omen. You will be elevated to a state of wealth and dignity.

Paradise: This is a very good dream. Hope of immortality and entrance into Paradise. Cessation of sorrows. Happy and healthy life.

Pigs: This indicates a mixture of good and bad luck. You will have great troubles but you will succeed. Many enemies are there, but there are some who will help you.

Prison: This is a dream of contrary. Indicates freedom and happiness.

Rain: This foretells trouble especially when it is heavy and boisterous. Gentle rain is a good dream indicating happy and calm life.

River: Rapid and flowing muddy river indicates great troubles and difficulties. But a river with calm glassy surface foretells happiness and love.

Ship: If you have a ship of your own sailing on the sea, it indicates advancement in riches. A ship that is tossed in the ocean and about to sink indicates disaster in life.

Singing: This is a dream of contrary. It indicates weeping and grief. Much suffering.

Snakes: You have sly and dangerous enemies who will injure your character and state of life.

Thunder: Great danger in life. Faithful friends will desert you. Thunder from a distance indicates that you will overcome troubles.

Volcano: Quarrels and disagreements in life.

Water: This indicates birth (of some person).

Wedding: This indicates that there is a funeral to be witnessed by you. To dream that you are married indicates that you will never marry. Marriage of sick persons indicates their death.

Young: To dream of young persons indicates enjoyment. If you are young, it indicates your sickness. You may die quickly.

www.ingramcontent.com/pod-product-compliance
Lightning Source LLC
Chambersburg PA
CBHW081259040426
42452CB00014B/2566

9 7 8 1 6 0 7 9 6 3 5 8 5